Hey Sis, Can We Talk?

Life-Changing Wisdom for Your Journey Through Your 20s

Destiny Pierce

Contents

Introduction

This book is a labor of love, a culmination of lessons learned, hardships endured, and wisdom gained from a life that began in the depths of a dysfunctional childhood that so many of us experience various degrees of. It is a guide, a beacon of hope, and a testament to the resilience of the human spirit. As a woman who has navigated the learning cycles that the turbulent waters of childhood trauma and abuse instinctively trigger to emerge with boundaries, self-love, and an unshakable sense of self, I write this not just as an author but as a sister, a mentor, and a guide.

You, my dear sisters in your late teens and twenties, stand at the threshold of life's many adventures and challenges. While some of you have been nurtured in functional homes, equipped with the tools and teachings for a smooth journey, many others have not been so fortunate. The disparity in what you have been taught, depending on the degree of functionality of your upbringing, is profound. This book aims to bridge that gap, to offer you the lessons and insights that a dysfunctional childhood did not.

My journey has been a testament to the fact that one can

climb out of the darkest pits of past trauma and transform pain into power. The signs from the universe have been unmistakable, guiding me to share my story and insights with you. Writing this book has crossed my mind many times and I even started writing it a few times, but this time was different. The Universe would not let me leave this book in my draft folder any longer. The morning after I began working on this book again, I woke up to Aaliyah's "If Your Girl Only Knew," magically cued up on my phone. I did not have a music streaming app opened on my phone. In fact, I rarely stream music from my phone and had not streamed music on my phone recently, so I was surprised to see a music app open in my notifications, but when I read the song title that was queued in the notifications, I immediately understood. It was the Universe's nudge to get me to this moment, where I pen down decades of experiences and realizations.

This book is more than just pages filled with words; it is a companion for your journey. Keep it close, in your pocketbook, purse, backpack, or nightstand. Let it be a constant reminder that you are not alone in your struggles, and that enlightenment, joy, and fulfillment are not just distant dreams but achievable realities.

Each chapter of this book addresses crucial aspects of life that you may have missed learning about if you grew up in a dysfunctional environment. From setting healthy boundaries to understanding the importance of rest and recovery, from navigating personal relationships to building a life of financial and emotional independence, this book covers it all.

My dear little sister, you are at a beautiful stage of life, full of potential and possibilities. It is my deepest hope that the lessons contained in these pages will empower you, illuminate your path, and help you avoid the unnecessary hardships and pains that life may throw your way. May you use this knowledge to live an enlightened life full of joy in your late teens and twenties.

With all my love and blessings,

Your Big Sis,

Destiny

Don't Take Everything Seriously

Embrace Lightness in Life

In life, we often shoulder burdens that aren't ours to carry, especially when our upbringing was clouded by chaos and confusion. In my 20s, I learned a hard lesson: not every decision is a matter of life or death. This realization is liberating. Understanding that you're only responsible for your own decisions, not those of your parents or peers, is crucial. It's about recognizing the fine line between what truly matters and the everyday choices that don't define our entire existence. Learning to differentiate these is key to finding peace and joy in the simplicity of life.

Three Steps To Take Today:

Mindful Reflection: Each evening, take a moment to reflect on your day. Identify instances where you might have overemphasized the gravity of a situation. Acknowledge these moments and gently remind yourself of the bigger picture.

Joyful Activities: Regularly engage in activities that bring you joy and laughter. Whether it's watching a comedy, spending time with friends who lift your spirits, or engaging in a hobby you love, make room for lightness in your daily life.

Affirmations of Release: Start your day with affirmations that encourage a lighter approach to life. Phrases like "Today, I choose to take things lightly" or "I am free from the weight of unnecessary burdens" can set a positive tone for your day.

Love Yourself the Most

Take the Journey to Genuine Self-Love

The path to self-love isn't a straight line, especially for those of us who grew up in dysfunctional families. Our early examples of 'love' often masked deeper issues, leaving us with a skewed understanding of what loving oneself truly means. This journey involves unlearning these misconceptions and peeling back the layers of our upbringing. True self-love emerges not as a sudden revelation but as a gradual acceptance and appreciation of self. It's a process of discovering and healing, leading to a place where self-care, boundaries, and peace become our nature.

Three Steps To Take Today:

Self-Care Routine: Establish a daily self-care routine that honors your body, mind, and spirit. This could be a skincare routine, a few minutes of meditation, or preparing a healthy meal for yourself.

Journaling for Self-Discovery: Keep a journal where you explore your feelings, dreams, and the steps you're taking towards loving yourself more. This practice encourages introspection and self-compassion.

Positive Self-Talk: Be mindful of your internal dialogue. Replace critical or negative thoughts with kind, loving words. Speak to yourself as you would to someone you love deeply. Start your day with a morning affirmation of "I am beautiful. I am gorgeous. I am smart."

Laugh at Yourself

Find Humor in Your Imperfection

One of the greatest gifts we can give ourselves is the ability to laugh at our mistakes. By laughing at ourselves, we take our power back. Growing up in an environment where every action was scrutinized or disproportionately punished, the fear of making mistakes can become deeply ingrained, but here's the truth: mistakes are an inevitable and essential part of life. They are not just missteps, but serve as opportunities for growth, learning and ensuring that our emotional maturity keeps pace with our physical maturity. Embracing our imperfections with humor is a powerful way to free ourselves from the chains of fear and to embrace a more compassionate and forgiving view of ourselves.

Three Steps To Take Today:

Reflect on Past Mistakes with Humor: Look back at past mistakes and find the humor in them. Recognize that these were learning experiences and allow yourself a light-hearted perspective on them.

Share Funny Stories: Share your embarrassing or funny moments with trusted friends or family. This not only lightens the mood but also helps normalize the idea of being imperfect.

Laughter Yoga or Therapy: Consider trying laughter yoga or laughter therapy sessions. These practices are designed to help you embrace joy and humor in everyday life.

Forgive Yourself – You're Doing Your Best

Give Yourself Grace on Your Journey

Forgiveness is often seen as something we extend to others, but self-forgiveness is just as vital. It's about acknowledging that we're doing our best with the knowledge and resources we have at any given moment. This kind of compassion towards ourselves is a crucial aspect of personal growth. It allows us to move forward with understanding and patience, recognizing that our journey is one of continuous learning and evolution.

Three Steps To Take Today:

Forgiveness Affirmations: Use affirmations focused on self-forgiveness, such as "I forgive myself for my past mistakes" or "I am learning and growing every day."

Reflective Writing: Write letters to yourself, expressing forgiveness for specific incidents or general feelings of guilt. It's a powerful way to release past burdens.

Seek Support: Sometimes, talking to a friend, family member, or therapist can help in the process of forgiving yourself. Sharing your feelings and receiving reassurance can be very healing. Just be sure that the person you choose to talk to can be trusted with your thoughts and feelings.

Create a Daily Self-Love Ritual

Cultivate a Practice of Self-Care

A daily self-love ritual is a powerful tool in reinforcing our commitment to ourselves. It can be as simple as a few moments of meditation, journaling, or engaging in personal grooming that uplifts our spirits. Such rituals are affirmations of our worth and our commitment to our well-being. They become a foundation for a life lived with intention, care, and love for oneself.

Three Steps To Take Today:

Daily Moments of Gratitude: Start or end your day by listing three things you are grateful for about yourself. This practice helps reinforce positive self-perception.

Personalize Your Space: Create a personal space in your home dedicated to self-love rituals, such as a meditation corner, reading nook, or a special chair for journaling.

Self-Love Dates: Schedule regular 'dates' with yourself where you do something that makes you feel happy and cherished, be it a solo movie night, a spa day, or a peaceful walk in nature.

It's Not You, It's Them (and It's Not Them, It's You)

Own Your Emotional Space

Navigating emotional turbulence is part of the human experience, but understanding that we're not responsible for others' emotions is crucial. When faced with anger or negativity from others, it's important to remember that these reactions are a reflection of their inner world, not ours. Owning our emotional space means recognizing our power to choose our responses and actions in order to maintain our inner peace regardless of external circumstances.

Three Steps To Take Today:

Emotional Awareness Practice: Regularly check in with your emotions. Identify what you're feeling and why, especially after interactions with others, to understand your emotional responses better.

Boundary Setting: Learn to set and enforce healthy boundaries. Politely but firmly assert your limits in relationships and interactions.

Mindfulness and Grounding Techniques: When you find yourself affected by others' emotions, use mindfulness or grounding techniques to bring yourself back to your own emotional center.

You Are Worthy!

Embrace Your Intrinsic Value

Every one of us is born with inherent worth. Our value doesn't come from external achievements or validation, but simply from our existence. This truth can sometimes be obscured by the challenges and experiences we face, particularly as children in a dysfunctional family setting. Recognizing and embracing our worth is a fundamental step towards living a life filled with joy, respect, and fulfillment. It's a powerful affirmation that guides us in making decisions that honor our true selves.

Three Steps To Take Today:

Daily Worthiness Reminders: Start your day by reminding yourself of your worth. A simple statement like "I am valuable and deserving of happiness" can set a positive tone for the day.

Recognize Your Achievements: Regularly acknowledge your achievements, no matter how small. Celebrating your successes reinforces your sense of self-worth.

Surround Yourself with Positivity: Choose to spend time with people and in environments that affirm your worth. Positive reinforcement from external sources can complement your internal beliefs.

Understand that Emotional Pain Leads to Physical Illness

The Mind-Body Connection

The connection between our emotional health and physical well-being is undeniable. Emotional pain, if left unaddressed, manifests in the body in various forms. From my journey, I've realized that many physical ailments are often rooted in unresolved emotional issues. It's essential to acknowledge and address these emotional pains to prevent them from impacting our physical health. Healing begins with understanding and accepting that our emotions and body are intricately linked. Disease is simply dis-ease in the body.

Three Steps To Take Today:

Emotional Awareness: Make it a habit to check in with your emotions regularly. Identifying and acknowledging your feelings is the first step in addressing them.

Seek Professional Help: If you're dealing with persistent emotional pain, consider seeking help from a therapist or counselor.

Mindfulness Practices: Engage in mindfulness practices like yoga or meditation, which can help in understanding and managing the connection between your emotional and physical health.

Learn to Regulate Your Emotions

Master Your Emotional Self-Regulation

Learning to regulate our emotions is a powerful skill. It doesn't mean suppressing our feelings but understanding them and responding in a way that aligns with our best selves. This skill is crucial in navigating life's ups and downs without being overwhelmed. Through my own experiences, I've learned that emotional regulation is about balance - acknowledging our emotions, understanding their origins, and then choosing how to express them in healthy ways.

Three Steps To Take Today:

Emotional Literacy: Work on identifying and naming your emotions. The better you can articulate what you feel, the easier it is to manage them.

Breathing Techniques: Practice breathing exercises. Deep breathing can be an effective tool in calming intense emotions.

Reflective Journaling: Keep a journal to reflect on your emotional responses to different situations. This can help in understanding patterns and triggers.

Heal Your Emotions, Heal Your Life

Take the Journey of Emotional Healing

Emotional healing is a transformative process that impacts every aspect of our lives. It involves delving into past wounds, understanding them, and actively working towards healing. This journey is not easy, but it's one of the most rewarding paths we can embark on. By healing our emotions, we open doors to new possibilities, healthier relationships, and a more fulfilling life. It's a process of reclaiming our power and finding peace within ourselves.

Three Steps To Take Today:

Self-Compassion: Practice self-compassion. Be gentle with yourself as you navigate your emotional healing journey.

Healing Activities: Engage in activities that promote healing, such as therapy, meditation, or art.

Support Network: Build a support network of friends, family, or support groups who understand and support your healing journey.

Forgive Others (But Don't Stick Around for Abuse)

Find Strength in Forgiveness

Forgiveness is not about condoning hurtful behavior; it's about freeing ourselves from the hold it has on our hearts. It's a gift we give ourselves. Forgiving others, especially in instances of abuse, is complex. While forgiveness can be healing, it's also essential to ensure that we are not exposing ourselves to further harm. Through my own experiences, I've learned that forgiveness is a process that takes time and is a part of the healing journey.

Three Steps To Take Today:

Understand Forgiveness: Reflect on the meaning of forgiveness and how it can be beneficial for your emotional well-being.

Set Boundaries: Forgiveness doesn't mean you have to stay in a harmful situation. Set clear boundaries to protect yourself.

Letting Go Rituals: Create rituals that symbolize letting go of the hurt, such as writing a letter (that you don't necessarily have to send) or a meditative practice.

A Mental Health Day is a Valid Reason to Call In

Honor Your Mental Well-being

Taking a mental health day is as crucial as taking a day off for physical illness. It's a recognition that our mental health is just as important as our physical health. In my life, I've learned the importance of listening to my mental and emotional needs and giving myself permission to rest. A mental health day can be a powerful tool in preventing burnout, reducing stress, and rejuvenating our minds.

Three Steps To Take Today:

Listen to Your Body and Mind: Be attentive to signs that you might need a break, such as feeling overwhelmed or fatigued.

Plan Your Mental Health Day: When taking a mental health day, have a plan on how you will spend it to ensure it's rejuvenating.

Communicate Clearly: If possible, communicate your need for a mental health day clearly and professionally to your employer or those affected.

Your Mindset Determines Your Reality

Shape Your Reality with Your Thoughts

Our mindset has a powerful impact on our reality. What we believe, how we think, and how we view the world shapes our experiences. Adopting a positive, growth-oriented mindset can transform challenges into opportunities and setbacks into learning experiences. Through my journey, I've embraced the power of positive thinking, not as a mere cliché, but as a tool for creating a fulfilling and meaningful life.

Three Steps To Take Today:

Positive Affirmations: Use positive affirmations to reinforce a growth mindset and shift negative thought patterns.

Mindful Awareness: Practice mindfulness to become aware of your thoughts and gently guide them towards positivity.

Learn from Challenges: View challenges as opportunities for growth. Reflect on what each experience can teach you.

Guilt and Shame are Wastes of Your Energy

Release the Burden of Guilt and Shame

Guilt and shame are emotions that can consume vast amounts of our energy and hinder our growth. They often stem from past experiences and internalized negative beliefs. Recognizing that these feelings do not define us is a crucial step in our journey to emotional freedom. Releasing guilt and shame involves understanding their roots, challenging the beliefs that fuel them, and actively choosing self-compassion and forgiveness.

Three Steps To Take Today:

Identify the Source: Reflect on what triggers feelings of guilt or shame. Understanding their origin is the first step in addressing them.

Challenge Negative Beliefs: Actively challenge and reframe the negative beliefs that contribute to your feelings of guilt and shame.

Practice Self-Compassion: Engage in self-compassion exercises, reminding yourself that you are deserving of love and forgiveness.

Cleanse Your Energy at Least Once a Day

Incorporate Some Form of Energy Cleansing

In the pursuit of wellness, we often overlook the subtlety of our energies. Cleansing your energy isn't just a spiritual practice; it's a necessary daily ritual for maintaining emotional and mental balance. I've experienced firsthand how a clouded energy field can lead to a clouded mind and life. Just like we cleanse our bodies, our energies too need regular cleansing to remove the negativity that accumulates daily. This practice brings clarity, peace, and a renewed sense of purpose.

Three Steps To Take Today:

Daily Meditation: Start or end your day with meditation. It helps in clearing the mind and resetting your energy.

Nature Walks: Spend time in nature. The natural environment has a way of cleansing and rejuvenating our energy fields.

Energy Cleansing Techniques: Learn and practice energy cleansing techniques such as using sage, visualization, or sound healing.

Good Dental Hygiene Keeps the Rest of Your Body Healthy

Dental Hygiene Impacts Overall Health

Dental health is more than just about having a bright smile; it's a window to your overall health. Neglecting oral care can lead to not just dental problems but also has been linked to heart disease, diabetes, and other health issues. From my own experience with oil pulling and making my own natural toothpaste, I've come to appreciate the profound impact of good oral hygiene on my overall health. It's an essential part of self-care that goes beyond aesthetics.

Three Steps To Take Today:

Regular Dental Check-Ups: Ensure regular visits to the dentist for professional cleanings and check-ups.

Daily Oral Hygiene Routine: Adopt a thorough daily oral hygiene routine including brushing, flossing, and using a mouthwash.

Explore Natural Methods: Consider incorporating natural oral care methods like oil pulling into your routine.

Everything in Your Body is Connected

Gain a Holistic View of Health

The interconnectedness of our body systems is a fundamental principle in understanding health. Recognizing that each part of our body impacts the other has been a cornerstone in my journey towards holistic wellness. When one system is out of balance, it can affect the whole body. This understanding encourages a more comprehensive approach to health, focusing on the entire body rather than just isolated symptoms or areas.

Three Steps To Take Today:

Holistic Health Practices: Engage in practices that promote holistic health, such as yoga or Tai Chi, which focus on the balance of mind, body, and spirit.

Balanced Diet: Eat a balanced diet that nourishes all parts of your body.

Mind-Body Connection: Pay attention to how your emotions affect your physical health and vice versa. Practice stress-reduction techniques to maintain this balance.

Learn About Your pH

Understand the Balance Within

In the grand tapestry of wellness and health, understanding the pH levels in our bodies is like discovering a hidden language of wellbeing. pH, which measures how acidic or alkaline our bodies are, is not just a concept confined to science laboratories; it's a significant aspect of our health. In my journey, particularly as I navigated the waters of holistic healing and wellness, the realization of how pH balance impacts our overall health was a revelation.

The body's pH balance is a fine line that determines so much of our health and well-being. When our pH levels are balanced, our bodies function optimally. But when they are off, it can lead to a host of health issues. Understanding your body's pH can provide insight into your overall health and guide you in making dietary and lifestyle choices that promote balance.

Three Steps To Take Today:

Educate Yourself: Learn about pH levels and their impact on the body. There are many resources available that explain how different foods and lifestyle choices can affect your body's pH.

Balance Your pH When Necessary: This product - N'More Boric Acid Vaginal Suppositories – is a must-have staple for your self-care cabinet. Keep this on hand at all times and use it whenever your body gives you the signal that you need to balance your pH.

Dietary Adjustments: Based on your findings, make dietary adjustments to help balance your pH. Incorporating more alkaline foods like fruits and vegetables can be beneficial.

Healthy Gut = Healthy Mind and Body

Embrace the Gut-Brain Connection

The health of our gut is intricately linked to the health of our mind and body. A healthy gut contributes to a strong immune system, improved mood, and effective digestion, among other benefits. Personally, adjusting my diet to nurture my gut health has had profound effects on my overall well-being. It's a testament to the fact that what we eat directly impacts our physical and mental health.

Three Steps To Take Today:

Probiotics and Prebiotics: Include foods rich in probiotics and prebiotics in your diet to support gut health.

Mindful Eating: Practice mindful eating to improve digestion and gut health.

Limit Harmful Foods: Reduce the intake of foods that can harm gut health, like processed foods and excessive sugar.

Nurture Your Energy Field (Aura)

Care for Your Aura

Our aura, or energy field, is an extension of our physical and emotional selves. Keeping this energy vibrant and clear is essential for our overall well-being. Personal experiences have taught me the importance of regularly nurturing my aura through various practices. This not only enhances my physical and emotional health but also improves my interactions with others.

Three Steps To Take Today:

Aura Cleansing Practices: Regularly engage in aura cleansing practices like meditation, spending time in nature, or using crystals.

Positive Surroundings: Surround yourself with positive people and environments, as these have a significant impact on your aura.

Self-Care Rituals: Incorporate self-care rituals like salt and herbal baths that not only nurture your body but also your energy field.

Limit Processed Foods

Incorporate Whole Foods Into Your Diet

The shift from processed to whole foods is a transformative journey for both the mind and body. Processed foods, while convenient and cheap, often come at the cost of our health, laden with additives and lacking in essential nutrients. Through my journey, I've learned that a diet rich in whole foods provides not just physical health benefits but also clarity of mind and energy. It's about making choices that honor our bodies' needs.

Three Steps To Take Today:

Meal Planning: Plan meals in advance to include a variety of whole foods and reduce reliance on processed foods.

Read Labels: Become adept at reading food labels to understand what you're consuming.

Cook at Home: Develop a habit of cooking at home, where you can control the ingredients and avoid processed elements.

Oil Pulling Eliminates Morning Breath and Face Break-Outs

Discover the Benefits of Oil Pulling

Oil pulling, an ancient practice, has been a revelation in my personal health regimen. This simple yet effective practice not only promotes oral health but also has surprising benefits for overall facial clarity. It's a testament to the power of natural and holistic health practices that often get overlooked in our modern lifestyles.

Three Steps To Take Today:

Regular Oil Pulling: Incorporate oil pulling into your daily morning routine.

Choose the Right Oil: Use high-quality oils like coconut or sesame oil and enhance with food grade essential oils for oil pulling.

Be Consistent: Consistency is key. Practice oil pulling regularly to see significant benefits.

Embrace Solitude

Your Strength is Found in Solitude

Solitude is not loneliness; it's a chosen moment of self-reflection and peace. In my life's journey, embracing solitude has been a powerful tool for self-discovery and growth. It's in these quiet moments that we truly listen to our inner voices and connect deeply with our core. Solitude allows us to recharge, to contemplate our life's path, and to emerge with a clearer, more focused mind. It's a sacred time to nurture our spirit and honor our individuality.

Three Steps To Take Today:

Schedule Time for Solitude: Actively set aside time in your schedule for solitude. It can be as simple as a few quiet moments in the morning or a solitary walk.

Create a Solitude Space: Designate a special place in your home where you can be alone with your thoughts, free from distractions.

Mindful Activities: Engage in activities that nurture your soul during your solitude, such as reading, journaling, or practicing mindfulness.

Explore Your Spirituality and Form a Connection with God

Develop a Personal Journey to Spiritual Connection

Exploring spirituality is a deeply personal journey, one that is unique to each individual. For me, forming a connection with God has been about understanding the divine presence in all aspects of life. It's about seeking a relationship with a higher power that guides, comforts, and gives purpose to our existence. This spiritual exploration is not just about religious practices; it's about finding a personal connection that resonates with your soul and enriches your life.

Three Steps To Take Today:

Spiritual Practices: Engage in spiritual practices that connect you to the divine. This could be prayer, meditation, or attending religious services.

Spiritual Reading: Read spiritual texts or literature that inspire and deepen your understanding of your faith and spirituality.

Reflective Time: Spend time in reflection, contemplating your beliefs and your relationship with the divine.

God is Real and is the Source of Your Life

Acknowledge the Divine Source

Believing in a higher power, in a divine force that is the source of all life, brings a profound sense of purpose and direction. My belief in God has been the foundation upon which I've built my life. It's a belief that offers comfort, guidance, and an understanding that we are part of something greater than ourselves. Recognizing this divine source in our lives brings a sense of peace and continuity amidst life's chaos.

Three Steps To Take Today:

Daily Devotionals: Dedicate time each day to connect with God through prayer, meditation, or reading spiritual texts.

Gratitude Practice: Regularly practice gratitude, acknowledging the divine presence in your blessings.

Nature Appreciation: Spend time in nature to feel closer to the divine creation and to reflect on the beauty and intricacy of life.

Mother-Father God Loves You Fully and Completely

Embrace Divine Love

The concept of a Mother-Father God is about embracing the divine as a source of unconditional love and nurturing. This belief has been a guiding light in my life, a reminder that we are loved and cherished beyond our understanding. It's a love that encompasses all aspects of our being and existence, a love that is constant and unwavering. Embracing this divine love is about accepting that we are valued, cared for, and an integral part of the universe.

Three Steps To Take Today:

Affirmations of Love: Regularly affirm to yourself that you are loved and cherished by the divine.

Journaling on Love: Write about your experiences and feelings of divine love, documenting how it manifests in your life.

Acts of Love: Engage in acts of kindness and love towards others, reflecting the divine love that you embrace.

Be in the Present Moment

Embrace the Power of Now

Living in the present moment is a practice that transforms our experience of life. So often, we are caught up in the regrets of the past or the anxieties of the future, missing the beauty and opportunities that the present moment offers. Being present has allowed me to appreciate life more fully, to engage with the world in a more meaningful way, and to find joy in the ordinary. It's about embracing life as it unfolds, one moment at a time.

Three Steps To Take Today:

Mindfulness Meditation: Practice mindfulness meditation to enhance your ability to live in the present moment.

Focused Activities: Engage in activities that require your full attention, helping you to stay present.

Mindful Reminders: Set reminders throughout your day to pause and bring your focus back to the present moment.

Ask for Guidance – on Both the Earth and Spiritual Planes

Seek Wisdom Beyond Ourselves

Asking for guidance, whether it's from people we trust on earth or from the spiritual realm, is an acknowledgment of our interconnectedness and the wisdom that surrounds us. In my journey, seeking guidance has been about humility and openness to learning from others and from the divine. It's about recognizing that we don't have all the answers and that there is profound wisdom in seeking help and guidance.

Three Steps To Take Today:

Seek Mentors: Identify and seek out mentors or advisors whom you respect and trust.

Spiritual Communication: Regularly communicate with the divine through prayer or meditation, asking for guidance and wisdom.

Openness to Learning: Maintain an attitude of openness and willingness to learn from various sources, both earthly and spiritual.

Pay Yourself First

Live by the Principle of Financial Self-Care

Paying yourself first is not just a financial strategy; it's an act of self-respect and foresight. I learned early in my career, even on a modest salary, the importance of setting aside a portion of my earnings for my future self. This approach not only prepared me for eventual financial independence but also instilled a sense of discipline and self-worth. It's about prioritizing your long-term financial well-being, ensuring that your future is as important as your present.

Three Steps To Take Today:

Automate Savings: Set up an automatic transfer to your savings account each time you get paid.

Budget Wisely: Create a budget that includes 'paying yourself first' as a non-negotiable expense.

Financial Goals: Set clear financial goals for your savings, whether it's retirement, an emergency fund, or a major purchase.

Take Your Vacation Days

Place Value on Your Rest and Rejuvenation

In our often relentless pursuit of career success, taking vacation days can seem like a luxury we can't afford. However, through my journey, I've realized the immense value of stepping away from work to rest and recharge. Vacation days are not just a perk; they're a necessity for maintaining balance, creativity, and long-term productivity. They offer a chance to reconnect with ourselves and our loved ones, to explore new places and ideas, and to return to our work with renewed energy and perspective.

Three Steps To Take Today:

Plan Your Vacations: Actively plan how you will use your vacation days each year.

Disconnect: During your vacation, truly disconnect from work to enjoy the time fully.

Balance Activities: Plan a mix of restful and active experiences during your vacations to maximize rejuvenation.

Use Your Sick Days

Honor Your Health and Well-being

Sick days are a crucial component of your employment benefits, meant to be used when your health and well-being demand it. Early in my career, I understood the importance of listening to my body and taking the time off when needed. It's a matter of self-care and acknowledging that your health is paramount. Using your sick days when necessary ensures that you can return to work with full strength and focus, ultimately benefiting both you and your employer.

Three Steps To Take Today:

Listen to Your Body: Be attentive to your body's signals and take a sick day when you're not feeling well.

Mental Health Matters: Remember that mental health is just as important as physical health. Take a sick day for mental health when needed.

Don't Feel Guilty: Release any guilt associated with taking sick days. Recognize that it's a responsible choice for your health and your job.

Create Your Own Cost-Benefit Decision Trees

Navigate Life's Choices with Clarity

A cost-benefit decision tree is a powerful tool for making informed, objective decisions. My own financial journey, including the decision to buy a house in my early 20s and retire by 45, was guided by weighing the costs and benefits of each major decision. This approach helps in visualizing the potential outcomes of our choices, ensuring that our decisions align with our long-term goals and values.

Three Steps To Take Today:

Learn Decision-Making Tools: Educate yourself on how to create and use a cost-benefit decision tree.

Apply It Regularly: Use this tool for both big and small decisions to develop a habit of thoughtful decision-making.

Review Your Decisions: Periodically review past decisions and their outcomes to refine your decision-making skills.

Value Your Time

Formalize the Currency of Your Life

Time is the most precious resource we have – it's the currency of life. Valuing your time means understanding your worth and choosing how and with whom you spend it wisely. Throughout my career, I've learned to assess opportunities not just in terms of financial gain but in terms of time investment as well. It's about prioritizing activities that align with your values, goals, and joy.

Three Steps To Take Today:

Time Audit: Regularly conduct a time audit to see where your time is going and adjust as needed.

Set Priorities: Clearly define your priorities and align your time investment with them.

Learn to Say No: Develop the skill of saying no to requests that don't align with your values or priorities.

Home Equity is a Great Way to Build Wealth

Invest in Your Future

Homeownership is not just about having a place to live; it's a strategic investment in your financial future. My decision to invest in a home right after college was a stepping stone to financial independence and early retirement. Building home equity is a tangible way to grow your wealth over time, offering both stability and the potential for significant financial gain.

Three Steps To Take Today:

Educate Yourself on Homeownership: Understand the process, benefits, and responsibilities of owning a home.

Financial Planning for Home Purchase: Start planning and saving for a home purchase as early as possible.

Long-Term Perspective: Consider your home as a long-term investment and make decisions accordingly.

Strive for Cash-Only Car (and Discretionary Spend) Purchases

Avoid the Debt Trap of Car Loans

Opting for cash-only car purchases is a financial strategy that can save you from the high-interest rates and long-term debt associated with car loans. My approach to financial management has always been to avoid unnecessary debt, and this includes how I choose to purchase vehicles. It's a practice that requires discipline and patience but ultimately leads to greater financial freedom and less stress.

Three Steps To Take Today:

Start a Car Savings Fund: Begin setting aside money in a dedicated savings account for your next car purchase.

Budget Wisely: Adjust your budget to prioritize saving for a car.

Research Affordable Options: When it's time to buy, research and choose a car that aligns with your savings, avoiding the temptation to overspend.

Use Your Credit Cards as a Precursor to Cash-Only

Use Credit Wisely

Using credit cards wisely can be a powerful financial strategy. The key is to use them as a tool, not a crutch. By paying off the full amount each month, I was able to build a strong credit score without accruing debt. This approach requires discipline and a clear understanding of your financial limits. It's about making credit cards work for you, not against you.

Three Steps To Take Today:

Disciplined Spending: Only charge what you can afford to pay off in full at the end of the month.

Track Your Expenses: Keep a close eye on your credit card spending to ensure it aligns with your budget.

Timely Payments: Set reminders to pay your credit card bill on time to avoid interest and late fees.

Never Get a Payday Loan or a Predatory Lending Loan

Avoid Financial Pitfalls

Payday loans and predatory lending schemes are dangerous traps that can lead to a cycle of debt and financial ruin. In my financial journey, avoiding these types of loans was crucial to maintaining financial health and independence. These loans may seem like a quick fix but often come with exorbitant interest rates and terms that exploit the borrower.

Three Steps To Take Today:

Emergency Fund: Build an emergency fund to avoid the need for high-interest loans in case of unexpected expenses.

Educate Yourself: Understand the risks associated with payday loans and predatory lending.

Seek Alternatives: If in need, explore alternative lending options like credit unions or small personal loans with reasonable terms.

Your Skills are Valuable; Decide if You Want to Use Them for a Side Hustle

Monetize Your Talents

Recognizing and valuing your skills can open doors to additional income streams through side hustles. My career journey included leveraging my skills outside of my primary job, which not only provided extra income but also personal fulfillment and growth. It's about seeing your skills as assets and finding creative ways to monetize them.

Three Steps To Take Today:

Skill Assessment: Take inventory of your skills and interests to identify potential side hustle opportunities.

Market Research: Research the market demand for your skills.

Start Small: Begin your side hustle on a small scale to manage it alongside your primary job.

Your Job Can Fire You With No Notice. You Should Have that Same Level of Loyalty to Them.

Practice Professional Pragmatism

In the professional world, loyalty is important, but so is pragmatism. Understanding that your employment can end suddenly is a reality that demands a proactive approach to your career. Always be prepared with a plan B, keep your skills updated, and maintain a professional network. This mindset is not about being disloyal; it's about being prepared and recognizing the business nature of employment.

Three Steps To Take Today:

Continuous Learning: Continuously update and expand your skills to stay relevant in the job market.

Network Building: Regularly invest time in building and maintaining a professional network.

Have a Backup Plan: Always have an updated resume and a clear idea of your next steps should your job situation change unexpectedly.

If You Hate Your Current Job, Find a New One and Then Quit

Create Your Path to Professional Fulfillment

Staying in a job you hate can be detrimental to your mental and emotional well-being. My decision to leave a job only after securing a new one was a strategic move that ensured financial stability while pursuing job satisfaction. It's about not settling for less and taking proactive steps towards a fulfilling career.

Three Steps To Take Today:

Career Exploration: Explore and identify what you want in your next job. What will make you happier or more fulfilled?

Active Job Search: Start looking for new opportunities while still employed.

Strategic Transition: Plan your transition carefully to ensure minimal financial and professional disruption.

Ask for What You Want.
Playing Small Results
in Receiving Small

Practice Your Power of Assertiveness

Asking for what you want in your career and in life is not just about negotiation; it's about recognizing your worth and believing in your abilities. In my early career, I learned the importance of this assertiveness, even on a limited salary. It's about setting your sights high and not being afraid to voice your ambitions and needs. Whether it's a raise, a new role, or more responsibilities, playing small often leads to being overlooked. Assertiveness is a skill that, when exercised with confidence and clarity, can lead to significant growth and opportunities.

Three Steps To Take Today:

Self-Reflection: Regularly assess your career goals and the steps needed to achieve them.

Skill Enhancement: Continuously improve your skills and knowledge to back up your requests with competence.

Effective Communication: Develop clear and assertive communication skills to articulate your desires and needs confidently.

Do Not Lend Money to Family or Friends

Navigate Financial Relationships with Wisdom

Lending money to family and friends can often lead to strained relationships and financial strain. Drawing from my personal experiences of financial discipline and decision-making, I understand the importance of maintaining healthy financial boundaries. If you are in a position to help, consider giving the amount as a gift rather than a loan. This approach eliminates the expectation of repayment and the potential for conflict. Financial generosity should come from a place of willingness and ability, not obligation or pressure.

Three Steps To Take Today:

Set Clear Boundaries: Clearly communicate your boundaries regarding lending money to family and friends.

Offer Alternatives: If you can't give money, offer other forms of support like advice or help in finding financial resources.

Financial Planning: Prioritize your financial security and goals. Only offer financial help if it doesn't compromise your financial wellbeing.

Get Clear About Your Boundaries

Be Clear about Personal Boundaries

Setting personal boundaries is a profound act of self-respect. It's about knowing your limits, your values, and what you are willing to accept in your relationships and life. In my journey, understanding and defining these boundaries has been central to maintaining not just my well-being but also my sense of self. It took purchasing my first home and navigating my career path to truly understand how clear boundaries set the tone for respectful and fulfilling interactions. Boundaries are not just lines drawn around us; they are statements of our self-worth.

Three Steps To Take Today:

Self-Reflection: Spend time reflecting on what you value, what you can tolerate, and what you cannot in your relationships.

Communicate Your Boundaries: Once you know your boundaries, communicate them clearly to those around you.

Re-evaluation: Regularly review and adjust your boundaries as your life and circumstances change.

Practice Enforcing Your Boundaries

Navigate the Art of Upholding Boundaries

Enforcing boundaries is not always easy, especially when it involves people we care about. However, it's an essential practice for preserving our integrity and well-being. Through my own experiences, including the challenges I faced in my early professional life, I learned that consistently upholding my boundaries was key to my growth and happiness. It's about respecting yourself enough to ensure others respect your boundaries too.

Three Steps To Take Today:

Consistency: Be consistent in enforcing your boundaries, regardless of the situation or person involved.

Assertive Communication: Develop the skill of assertively communicating your boundaries without being aggressive.

Support System: Build a support system of friends or mentors who respect your boundaries and encourage you to maintain them.

Make No Exceptions When It Comes to Your Boundaries

Be Unwavering in Your Standards

Making exceptions to our boundaries can often lead us down a path of compromise and disappointment. In my own life, particularly in my journey to financial independence, I recognized that making no exceptions in my boundaries was crucial for my success and peace of mind. It's a testament to your commitment to your values and self-respect. Boundaries are not negotiable; they are the foundations upon which healthy relationships and self-esteem are built.

Three Steps To Take Today:

Firmness in Decision-Making: Be firm and clear in your decisions that relate to your boundaries.

Reminders of Your Worth: Regularly remind yourself of your worth and why your boundaries are important.

Avoid Rationalizing: Avoid making excuses for others' behavior that crosses your boundaries.

Say No When You Mean No

Enjoy Your Power of a Respectful Decline

Saying 'no' is a powerful tool in maintaining our boundaries and integrity. It's about honoring your feelings, capacity, and priorities. In my path to early retirement, I realized that saying no to things that didn't align with my goals or values was just as important as saying yes to opportunities. It's about being true to yourself and not overcommitting or pleasing others at your expense.

Three Steps To Take Today:

Reflect Before Responding: Take time to consider requests before responding. Ensure your response aligns with your boundaries and priorities.

Polite but Firm Responses: Learn to say no in a way that is polite but firm, leaving no room for misunderstanding.

Guilt-Free Mindset: Remind yourself that it's okay to say no, and you shouldn't feel guilty for prioritizing your needs and boundaries.

Say Yes When You Mean Yes

Embrace Opportunities with Conviction

Saying 'yes' when you truly mean it is just as important as saying no. It's about embracing opportunities that align with your values and goals. In my journey, especially when making bold moves like buying a house early in my career, saying yes was about embracing opportunities that aligned with my long-term vision. It's a celebration of the things that bring us growth, joy, and fulfillment.

Three Steps To Take Today:

Identify Opportunities: Be open to opportunities that align with your values and goals.

Trust Your Instincts: Trust your instincts when an opportunity feels right.

Take Calculated Risks: Don't be afraid to take calculated risks that can lead to personal growth and achievement.

Don't Choose People Based on Their Potential

Value People for Who They Are Now

Choosing people based on their potential rather than their current reality can lead to disappointment and strained relationships. In my life, especially in my interactions and decisions on my path to retirement, I learned the importance of seeing and accepting people as they are. It's about forming relationships based on reality, not on what we hope someone will become.

Three Steps To Take Today:

Realistic Expectations: Set realistic expectations in your relationships.

Acceptance: Learn to accept people as they are, not as you wish them to be.

Self-Reflection: Reflect on why you may be inclined to choose people based on potential and how it impacts your relationships.

All Skin-Folk Ain't Kin-Folk and All Relatives are Not Family

Understand the Depth of Relationships

The saying 'all skin-folk ain't kin-folk and all relatives are not family' speaks to the truth that not all people who share our heritage or bloodline will necessarily have our best interests at heart. This realization, which became evident in my journey towards financial independence, is about recognizing that true kinship and family are defined by respect, support, and love, not just by biological or cultural ties.

Three Steps To Take Today:

Evaluate Relationships: Take time to evaluate your relationships based on mutual respect and support.

Cultivate Meaningful Connections: Focus on cultivating relationships with people who genuinely care for and support you.

Set Boundaries: Set clear boundaries in relationships that do not positively contribute to your well-being.

Your Co-Workers are Not Your Friends, Do Not Trust Them

Navigate Professional Relationships with Prudence

The professional world has its own set of dynamics, and it's important to navigate it with caution and prudence. The distinction between colleagues and friends is crucial. While friendly relationships at work are important, maintaining a certain level of professionalism and boundary is key. In my career, keeping this distinction clear was important in maintaining my focus on my goals, including early retirement, without getting entangled in potential workplace dramas or conflicts.

Three Steps To Take Today:

Maintain Professional Boundaries: Keep a healthy balance between being friendly and maintaining professional boundaries.

Discreet Sharing: Be discreet about what personal information you share in the workplace.

Develop Outside Friendships: Cultivate friendships outside of work to have a support system that is separate from your professional life.

Figure Out What You're Interested In and Explore It

Embrace Your Passions

Discovering and pursuing your interests is a journey towards self-fulfillment and joy. In my own life, from buying my first home to retiring early, following my interests has always been a guiding light. It's about listening to your heart and giving yourself the freedom to explore what truly excites you. Whether it's a hobby, a field of study, or a new skill, delving into your interests enriches your life, broadens your horizons, and often leads to unexpected opportunities.

Three Steps To Take Today:

Self-Exploration: Dedicate time to self-exploration to identify your interests.

Take Action: Once you identify an interest, take small steps towards exploring it, such as joining a class or reading related books.

Stay Open-Minded: Remain open to new experiences and be willing to adjust your path as you discover more about your interests.

There's an Herb for That!

Explore the Power of Natural Remedies

Incorporating natural remedies, like herbs, into your life is not just about treating ailments; it's a philosophy of living in harmony with nature. During my journey, exploring natural remedies was a part of embracing a holistic approach to health and well-being. It's about understanding the healing properties of plants and using them to support your body's natural healing processes. This approach fosters a deeper connection with nature and an appreciation for its gifts.

Three Steps To Take Today:

Educate Yourself: Learn about different herbs and their benefits.

Consult a Professional: Before using herbal remedies, consult with a healthcare professional, especially if you have existing health conditions.

Experiment Carefully: Start incorporating herbs into your life in small ways, like herbal teas or cooking, and observe their effects.

Everything You Feel Is a Signal

Understand the Language of Energy

Our emotions are powerful energetic signals that communicate our needs, fears, joys, and pains. In my path to personal and financial success, understanding and honoring my emotions was crucial. It's about recognizing that every emotion has a purpose and a message. By tuning into these signals, we can make more informed decisions, develop deeper self-awareness, and navigate life's challenges with greater clarity and wisdom.

Three Steps To Take Today:

Emotional Awareness: Regularly check in with yourself to identify and understand your emotions.

Journaling: Use journaling as a tool to process and reflect on your emotions.

Seek Understanding: Try to find the root cause of your emotions and what they are signaling about your needs or situation.

Stop the Self-Sabotage

Overcome Inner Obstacles

Self-sabotage is a barrier many of us face, often unknowingly. It's a pattern of behavior that hinders our progress and fulfillment. In my journey, recognizing and addressing my self-sabotaging behaviors was essential for achieving my goals, like early retirement. It's about identifying the ways in which we hold ourselves back and consciously working to change those patterns.

Three Steps To Take Today:

Identify Patterns: Reflect on past instances where you might have sabotaged your efforts and identify patterns.

Positive Affirmations: Use positive affirmations to counter negative self-talk and beliefs.

Seek Support: Consider seeking help from a counselor or coach to work through self-sabotaging behaviors.

Do Not Overshare

Perfect The Wisdom of Measured Sharing

Oversharing personal information can leave us vulnerable and often leads to uncomfortable situations. In my professional and personal life, I've learned the value of discretion. It's about sharing appropriately, considering the context and the relationship. This approach protects your privacy and fosters more meaningful and trustworthy connections.

Three Steps To Take Today:

Assess the Situation: Before sharing, assess the situation and the level of trust you have with the people involved.

Practice Discretion: Develop a habit of pausing and thinking before you speak, especially in new or informal settings.

Set Sharing Boundaries: Define clear boundaries for yourself about what you are comfortable sharing and with whom.

People Who Attack You Are Hurting and Often Jealous

Use Compassion in the Face of Negativity

Understanding that people who attack or criticize you are often projecting their own pain and insecurities can change how you respond to them. In my life, this understanding has been key to maintaining my peace and not taking things personally. It's about responding with compassion rather than defensiveness and recognizing the pain behind their actions.

Three Steps To Take Today:

Empathetic Response: Try to respond with empathy and understanding, rather than anger or defensiveness.

Maintain Boundaries: Protect yourself by maintaining strong boundaries with people who are consistently negative or hurtful.

Self-Care: After negative encounters, practice self-care to restore your balance and peace.

Make Plans Based on What You Know Today

Embrace the Present in Planning

Making plans based on your current reality, rather than waiting for an ideal future, is a pragmatic approach to life. It's about taking action now, with what you have and where you are. In my journey, this approach allowed me to seize opportunities and make progress towards my goals, like buying a house on a modest salary. It's a balance of planning for the future while being grounded in the present.

Three Steps To Take Today:

Realistic Goal Setting: Set goals based on your current situation and resources.

Action-Oriented Approach: Take actionable steps now, even if they are small, towards your goals.

Flexible Planning: Be flexible in your plans and open to adjusting them as your situation changes.

Do It Alone Until You Can Do It with the Right People

Find Your Strength in Solo Ventures

Sometimes, pursuing your goals alone is more effective than waiting for the right team or partner. In my life, particularly in my early career and financial decisions, I learned the value of self-reliance. It's about trusting your abilities and taking initiative, knowing that the right people will join you when the time is right. This approach fosters independence, confidence, and a deep sense of accomplishment.

Three Steps To Take Today:

Self-Confidence: Build confidence in your abilities to pursue goals independently.

Seek Knowledge: Educate yourself and acquire the necessary skills to achieve your goals.

Openness to Collaboration: Be open to collaboration in the future, but don't let the absence of it hold you back now.

The Lesson Will Repeat Until You Learn the Lesson

Embrace Life's Teachings

Life has a way of presenting us with the same challenges until we learn the lessons they offer. Recognizing this pattern was crucial in my journey towards personal and financial freedom. It's about understanding the underlying messages in repeated challenges and actively working to learn from them. This process is a powerful tool for personal growth and transformation.

Three Steps To Take Today:

Reflect on Patterns: Take time to reflect on recurring issues or challenges in your life.

Seek the Lesson: Try to identify the lesson or message in these repeated patterns.

Conscious Change: Actively work on making changes based on the lessons you identify.

Develop a Good Hygiene Routine

Create Your Foundation of Self-Care

A good hygiene routine is fundamental to not just physical health but also self-respect and confidence. In my life, maintaining a consistent hygiene routine was part of a broader commitment to self-care and well-being. It's a daily practice that says you value and care for yourself, contributing to a positive self-image and overall health.

Three Steps To Take Today:

Establish a Routine: Create and stick to a daily hygiene routine.

Personalize Your Care: Tailor your hygiene routine to your specific needs and preferences.

Regular Check-Ups: Include regular dental and medical check-ups in your routine for overall health maintenance.

You Are a Target If You Aren't Paying Attention

Know The Importance of Awareness and Vigilance

Staying aware and vigilant in both your personal and professional life is crucial for safety and success. My journey, especially in achieving financial independence, taught me the importance of being alert to potential risks and opportunities. It's about being conscious of your surroundings, the people you interact with, and the information you share, which helps in making informed decisions and protecting yourself from potential harm.

Three Steps To Take Today:

Stay Informed: Keep yourself informed about current events and trends, especially those relevant to your safety and well-being.

Mindfulness Practice: Practice mindfulness to enhance your awareness of your surroundings and interactions.

Protect Personal Information: Be cautious about the amount and type of personal information you share, especially in public and online.

Fix Problems Before They Fester

Prevent Escalation Through Early Resolution

Addressing problems early on, before they grow and fester, is essential for maintaining emotional and mental health. In my path to self-healing, recognizing and addressing issues promptly was crucial to prevent them from escalating. It's about being proactive in facing challenges, whether they're personal, professional, or emotional.

Three Steps To Take Today:

Mindful Awareness: Be mindful and aware of any emerging problems in your life.

Prompt Action: Take prompt action to address issues, seeking help when needed.

Regular Check-Ins: Regularly check in with yourself to identify and address any areas of concern.

Love Does Not Hurt

Recognize Healthy Love

Understanding that true love is nurturing, supportive, and respectful is fundamental to building healthy relationships. My experiences, both personally and professionally, taught me that love should not be painful or diminishing. Love is about mutual respect, growth, and support. It uplifts rather than tears down.

Three Steps To Take Today:

Define Love for Yourself: Reflect on what love means to you and what it looks like in practice.

Set Relationship Standards: Set clear standards for how you wish to be treated in relationships.

Healthy Relationship Models: Seek out and learn from healthy relationship models, whether through books, mentors, or therapy.

If You Grew Up in a Dysfunctional Home, Your Guidance System Will Be Screwed Up Until You Heal Yourself

Realign Your Internal Compass

Growing up in a dysfunctional home often leads to a skewed internal guidance system. Recognizing this was key in my journey towards healing and self-improvement. It's about understanding that the coping mechanisms and beliefs developed in such an environment may not serve us well in adulthood. Healing involves reassessing and realigning our internal guidance system to better suit our true selves and aspirations.

Three Steps To Take Today:

Self-Reflection: Reflect on how your upbringing has influenced your beliefs and decisions.

Seek Professional Help: Consider therapy or energy healing to help realign your internal guidance system.

Continuous Learning: Commit to continuous learning and self-improvement to overcome the limitations of your past environment.

It's More Important to Like Yourself Than to Be Liked by Others

Value Self-Acceptance

Valuing your own opinion of yourself over others' is a powerful stance in life. In my journey, learning to like and accept myself was integral to my well-being and success. It's about building self-esteem and self-love, understanding that seeking validation from others is a path to disappointment. True contentment and strength come from self-acceptance and self-appreciation.

Three Steps To Take Today:

Practice Self-Love: Regularly engage in acts of self-love and self-care.

Positive Self-Talk: Cultivate a habit of positive self-talk and affirmations.

Reduce Comparison: Actively work to reduce comparing yourself to others and focus on your own journey.

Accept the Experience and Move On

Embrace Life's Lessons and Moving Forward

Life is a mosaic of experiences, some exhilarating and some challenging. Accepting these experiences, learning from them, and then moving forward is a powerful practice. During my journey, from making bold financial decisions to personal development, embracing and accepting life's varied experiences was integral to my growth. It's about understanding that every experience, good or bad, brings wisdom and strength. Acceptance doesn't mean resignation; it means acknowledging the reality of a situation and then using it as a stepping stone to move forward.

Three Steps To Take Today:

Reflective Practice: Reflect on your experiences, focusing on the lessons they offer.

Acceptance Exercises: Engage in acceptance exercises, like mindfulness or journaling, to help process and accept your experiences.

Future Focus: After accepting an experience, shift your focus to the future and what positive steps you can take next.